Suljo Kunić
Amela Kunić
Emir Tupković

Electroneurographic parameters in patients with metabolic syndrome

Suljo Kunić
Amela Kunić
Emir Tupković

Electroneurographic parameters in patients with metabolic syndrome

LAP LAMBERT Academic Publishing

Impressum / Imprint

Bibliografische Information der Deutschen Nationalbibliothek: Die Deutsche Nationalbibliothek verzeichnet diese Publikation in der Deutschen Nationalbibliografie; detaillierte bibliografische Daten sind im Internet über http://dnb.d-nb.de abrufbar.
Alle in diesem Buch genannten Marken und Produktnamen unterliegen warenzeichen-, marken- oder patentrechtlichem Schutz bzw. sind Warenzeichen oder eingetragene Warenzeichen der jeweiligen Inhaber. Die Wiedergabe von Marken, Produktnamen, Gebrauchsnamen, Handelsnamen, Warenbezeichnungen u.s.w. in diesem Werk berechtigt auch ohne besondere Kennzeichnung nicht zu der Annahme, dass solche Namen im Sinne der Warenzeichen- und Markenschutzgesetzgebung als frei zu betrachten wären und daher von jedermann benutzt werden dürften.

Bibliographic information published by the Deutsche Nationalbibliothek: The Deutsche Nationalbibliothek lists this publication in the Deutsche Nationalbibliografie; detailed bibliographic data are available in the Internet at http://dnb.d-nb.de.
Any brand names and product names mentioned in this book are subject to trademark, brand or patent protection and are trademarks or registered trademarks of their respective holders. The use of brand names, product names, common names, trade names, product descriptions etc. even without a particular marking in this work is in no way to be construed to mean that such names may be regarded as unrestricted in respect of trademark and brand protection legislation and could thus be used by anyone.

Coverbild / Cover image: www.ingimage.com

Verlag / Publisher:
LAP LAMBERT Academic Publishing
ist ein Imprint der / is a trademark of
OmniScriptum GmbH & Co. KG
Heinrich-Böcking-Str. 6-8, 66121 Saarbrücken, Deutschland / Germany
Email: info@lap-publishing.com

Herstellung: siehe letzte Seite /
Printed at: see last page
ISBN: 978-3-8484-3558-6

Contents

1. Introduction

1.1. Metabolic syndrome

Metabolic syndrome is a cluster of disorders that includes central obesity, elevated blood pressure, increased triglycerides, decreased concentrations of high density lipoprotein and insensitivity to insulin. More recently, this list includes hypercoagulability, hyperuricemia and microalbuminuria.

Testimony of the existence of elements of the metabolic syndrome can be found on the sculptures of ancient civilizations as well as many paintings. Obesity was previously considered primarily an aesthetic problem, and in some cultures represented the ideal of beauty or a sign of belonging to the social elite.

Warnings on the dangerous merging of several risk factors (eng. *clustering*) started to appear during the last century, which has in recent years become especially important. Already Kylin (1923) pointed to the unfavorable combination of hypertension, hyperglycemia and hyperuricemia. Vague (1947) draws attention to the harmful effects of androgen type of obesity on metabolism of sugars and lipids, and Avogadro et al. (1967) point to a dangerous combination of obesity, diabetes and hyperlipoproteinaemia. Reaven (1988) argues that in the core of what is called "syndrome X" is insulin resistance. From the moment of its publication and, in the medical literature, in an attempt to differentiate between hyperinsulinemia and insulin resistance, some authors introduce alternative terms: *metabolic syndrome, dysmetabolic syndrome, cardiovascular dysmetabolic syndrome, plurimetabolic syndrome, insulin resistance syndrome, deadly quartet*, etc. The foundation of all of them is grounded in providing personal lists of variables that show a statistically different level of association with insulin resistance (Jarrett, 1998; Groop and Orho-Melander, 2001; Fagan and Deedwania, 1998).

1

The latest definition of the metabolic syndrome include a variety of metabolic disorders associated with the condition of insulin resistance, which is often associated with a high risk of the phenotype of above-average body mass and obesity.

There are three assumed etiologies of metabolic syndrome. The first is obesity, which is, as it turns out, responsible for the excessive release of free fatty acids, cytokines and other proinflammatory products that have been implicated in the development of insulin resistance, hypertension and dyslipidemia. Insulin resistance as another possible cause of metabolic syndrome is more or less represented in all categories of the increased body mass index. The third etiology includes independent factors: immune factors, vascular factors, liver factors, etc., which are influenced by specific individual genetic background and environmental factors (Grundy et al., 2004).

Criteria for diagnosis of metabolic syndrome are quite different among professional societies. The clinical definition of the International Federation of Diabetes (IDF) in 2005, is based on the presence of abdominal obesity defined by waist ≥ 94 cm for men and ≥ 80cm for women in Europe, and two of the remaining four criteria (Alberti et al., 2005):

- high triglycerides ≥ 1.7mmol / l, or previously treated abnormality;
- reduced levels of high density lipoprotein: ≤ 1.03mmol / l for men, and ≤ 1.29 mmol / l for women; or previously treated abnormality;
- elevated blood pressure: systolic ≥ 130 mmHg and / or diastolic ≥ 85 mm Hg; or previously treated hypertension;
- elevated levels of fasting glucose: ≥ 5.6 mmol / l; or pre-existing diabetes mellitus type 2

According to the guidelines of the National Cholesterol Education Program - Adult Treatment Panel III (NCEP-ATP III), obesity is taken as the most important criterion for the diagnosis of metabolic syndrome, defined by waist > 102 cm for men and > 88 cm for women. Other components that constitute the metabolic syndrome are:

- dyslipidemia (triglyceride ≥ 1.69 mmol / l or the concentration of high-density lipoprotein ≤ 1.04 mmol / l for men and ≤ 1.29 mmol / l for women);
- elevated arterial pressure (systolic ≥ 130 mm Hg, or diastolic ≥ 85 mm Hg) and
- elevated blood sugar (glucose concentration in the blood glucose ≥ 6.1 mmol / l; modified to ≥ 5.6 mmol / l in 2004).

Three or more positive criteria, i.e. two or more positive criteria with presence of obesity as defined by the waist size, are sufficient for diagnosis of metabolic syndrome (Anonymous, 2001; Deen, 2004; Anonymous, 2005).

The World Health Organization (WHO) recommended in 1999 the definition of metabolic syndrome through four components:

- arterial hypertension (antihypertensive treatment already in progress and/or increased arterial pressure, systolic ≥ 140 mm Hg or diastolic ≥ 90 mm Hg);
- dyslipidemia (triglyceride ≥ 1.7 mmol / l and/or concentration of high density lipoprotein < 0.9 mmol/l for men and < 0.85 mmol/l for women);
- obesity (body mass index ≥ 30kg/m² and/or waist to hip ratio > 0.90 for men and > 0.85 for women) and
- microalbuminuria (renal excretion of albumin ≥ 20 µg/min).

For the diagnosis of metabolic syndrome two or more positive criteria are needed, along with insulin resistance (hyperinsulinemia, fasting hyperglycemia or impaired glucose tolerance) (Anonymous, 1999).

Insulin resistance represents a state in which in addition to sustained, and even increased secretion of pancreas, insulin can not realize its cellular effects. Partially, circulating antagonists (e.g. cortisol, glucagon, etc.) can be blamed, as well as insulin antibodies, and the most important place is held by the receptor and postreceptor tissue deflection, resulting in a reduction of the effect of insulin (Smirčić-Duvnjak, 2004).

It was found that several growth factors and cytokines can modulate signaling of the insulin postreceptors. While insulin-like growth factor 1 (IGF-1) increases the activity of insulin-mediated cellular receptor, free fatty acids (FFA), tumor necrosis factor-alpha (TNF-α), and leptin, have the opposite effect (Douahue et al., 1999).

The research of pathophysiological mechanisms in the development of metabolic syndrome have shown that an increase in the levels of pro-inflammatory cytokines and TNF-α in plasma and tissues, may be the result of both inflammatory and emotional distress, which, as a consequence, has insulin resistance (Hristova and Aloe, 2006).

The gold standard in the diagnosis of insulin resistance is the so-called hyperinsulinaemic euglycaemic clamp: insulin is administered at a steady rate of infusion and glucose is maintained at basal levels through glucose infusion. The rate of glucose infusion provides a measure of glucose uptake in all tissues (DeFronzo et al., 1979).

Another, more convenient way is an indirect estimate of insulin resistance based on the index obtained from the results of oral glucose tolerance test (OGTT) which consists of measuring the concentration of fasting blood glucose, and testing the levels again, 120 minutes after the glucose load (75g glucose in 300ml water orally). It turned out that the results correlate well with the results of hyperinsulinemic euglycemic clamps. Several formulas have been developed that estimate insulin resistance in that way (Kanauchi, 2002; Stumvoll et al., 2000; Matsuda and DeFronzo, 1999).

Obesity represents excessive accumulation of fat in the body, most often defined by waist size or body mass index.

Every person has a genetically determined weight structure in which the body weight is strictly regulated by the energy homeostatic mechanism (Cummings and Schwartz, 2003; Bell et al., 2005; Korner and Leibel, 2003). In the pathophysiology of obesity, genetic background accounts for 40-80% (Bell et al., 2005), and so far at least 204 genetic loci associated with obesity have been identified. Some of them have been confirmed in several studies (Perusse et al., 2005).

Adipocytes of fat tissue secrete leptin and β-cells of the pancreas secrete insulin, both in proportion to body fat content. These two hormones enter the brain, bind to their receptors on the neurons of the hypothalamus and act to reduce body weight. Hypothalamic neurons express peptides and their receptors, which can be classified into two groups. The first group is called orexigens and it includes: neuropeptide Y, agouti-related protein (AgRP), melanin concentrating hormone (MCH), orexin A and B. The second group are anorexigenics: melanocortin, i.e. the melanocyte-stimulating hormone (MSH), and cocaine and amphetamine related transcript (CART). In a situation of increased serum concentrations of leptin or insulin anorexigenic pathways prevail, resulting in: an increase in energy consumption, an increase in thermogenesis and a decrease in food intake. Reduced serum concentrations of leptin and insulin induce activation of orexigenic pathways, leading to: a low rate of metabolism, and increased appetite. Leptin and insulin mediate in the long-term regulation of body weight, but they are also functional when it comes to short-term signals which begin or end individual meals (Cummings and Schwartz, 2003).

Food intake was also monitored in some other short-acting hormones/factors: ghrelin, motilin, neuromedin U, neurotensin (Nogueiras et al., 2005), cholecystokinin, peptide YY_{3-36} (Korner and Leibel, 2003) and glucagon-like peptide-1 (GLP-1) (King, 2005). All these hormones are secreted in the gastrointestinal tract, and through vagal afferent signaling (King, 2005). Ghrelin is secreted at the base of the stomach and increases the feeling of hunger and stimulates gastric emptying (Nogueiras et al., 2005), and PYY_{3-36} signals satiety and suppresses intestinal motility (Korner and Leibel, 2003).

The body's ability to precisely maintain body weight is reflected in the failure of interventions designed to reduce body weight. Diets with limited calories lead to a compensatory increase in the levels of ghrelin, which stimulates food intake (Korner and Leibel, 2003).

Since the observed positive correlation between insulin resistance and mass of visceral fat (Grundy et al., 2004), obesity is preferably classified according to the distribution, and not only to the amount of body fat. According to the distribution of body fat, there are two basic types of obesity: ginoid or female (pear-shaped) and android or male (apple shape). In gynoid obesity excess fat accumulates under the skin in the lower parts of the body, around the pelvis and thighs. These people have shown a higher susceptibility to mechanical complications in the form of complications of movement, insufficiency of peripheral venous circulation and respiratory insufficiency. This type of obesity may be present in both sexes. The android type (central or visceral type) is marked by the fat building up in the shoulders, chest and abdomen. This type of obesity has increased risk of cardiovascular and metabolic complications, as well as some forms of cancer (Bell et al., 2005).

Visceral and subcutaneous adipose tissue also differ according to their endocrine activities. Specific receptors such as receptors type 1 angiotensin II, b_1-, b_2- and b_3- adrenergic receptors, receptors for glucocorticoids and androgens, are represented to a greater extent in visceral adipose tissue, which promotes lipolysis (Kershaw and Flier, 2004; Vohl et al., 2004; Arner, 1995). Antilipolytic insulin receptors, α-2 adrenergic receptors and estrogen receptors predominate in the subcutaneous adipose tissue (Vohl et al., 2004; Arner, 1995). Visceral adipose tissue secretes its products into the portal circulation, causing the increase in the concentration of free fatty acids in the liver, where they then favor gluconeogenesis, synthesis of very low density lipoproteins and decrease glucose uptake, thus assisting in the development of insulin resistance. Visceral adipose tissue is characterized by relatively high secretion of interleukin 1 (IL-1) and plasminogen activator inhibitor 1 (PAI-1), while the secretion of leptin and adiponectin is greater in subcutaneous adipose tissue (Kershaw and Flier, 2004).

In obese subjects, the concentrations of soluble leptin receptors are low, and thus the fractions of bound leptin concentrations. This feature is associated with abdominal obesity and insulin resistance. It is believed that soluble leptin receptors play an important role in the transmission of the blood-brain barrier, and to transfer this saturation or distortion in the signal converting leptin receptor may be the cause of the so-called leptin resistance or desensitization (Meier and Gressner, 2004). In obese individuals, plasma leptin concentrations are elevated and exogenous administration of leptin has no effect on body weight (Kershaw and Flier, 2004). Along with this, leptin concentrations in cerebrospinal fluid are only slightly elevated (Meier and Gressner, 2004).

Lipids or fats are the compounds of various composition, and, as a rule, they are insoluble in water but soluble in organic solvents. Biologically, they are very important compounds. They are the main component of biological membranes and they affect their permeability, participate in the transfer of nerve impulses, create contacts between cells, make up energy reserves, protect the body from mechanical injury and form a thermal insulation layer (Clayden et al., 2001; David et al., 2005).

Since insoluble in water, in order to be transported through the bloodstream lipids bind to proteins, thus building lipoproteins. Given the density of lipid and protein complex, the following are distinguished:

- chylomicrons, which are the largest in diameter and have the lowest density (and the highest content of triglycerides),
- very low density lipoproteins (VLDL);
- intermediate (transitional) density lipoproteins (IDL);
- low density lipoproteins (LDL) and
- high density lipoproteins (HDL).

Dyslipidemia, as one of the components of the metabolic syndrome, is a complex process in which a change in the concentration of lipids in the body occurs. In this syndrome, it usually involves: elevated triglycerides, reduced high-density lipoprotein concentrations and elevated level of free fatty acids.

Increased carbohydrate intake (> 57% of the total energy needs of the body) causes a reduction in the level of high density lipoproteins and an increase in the concentration of triglycerides (Yang et al., 2002).

Arterial pressure is the force with which the circulating blood works on a unit of the area of the blood vessel, which is due to the contraction of cardiac muscle and the consequent movement of blood through the cardiovascular system. From the standpoint of physics, level of blood pressure (P) depends on the stroke volume of blood from the left ventricle (Q) and peripheral resistance in blood vessels (R), which can be represented using the formula: $P = Q \times R$.

In healthy subjects insulin stimulates the sympathetic nervous system that affects the blood vessels, causing vasodilation. Insulin also stimulates the reabsorption of sodium in the kidneys. In a state of insulin resistance vasodilatation can be lost, but the effect on the kidneys and sympathetic stimulation are maintained, even increased. These two effects both contribute to hypertension or a state of permanent high blood pressure. Hypertension additionally stimulates an increase in free fatty acids which again favor vasoconstriction. However, it seems that events associated directly with insulin resistance have only a moderate role in the development of hypertension (Eckel et al., 2005).

It was also found that leptin itself may to some extent contribute to hypertension, because the plasma concentrations of leptin-related protein in normotensive men correlate with sympathetic nervous activity (Tank et al., 2003).

Although about fifty different reasons for high blood pressure have been described to date (renal artery stenosis, polycystic kidney disease, hyperaldosteronism, Cuhing syndrome, atrio-ventricular fistula and other similar causes), these secondary forms can explain only about 5% of cases of the disease, and in all the others, the so called essential hypertension is the cause, for which the exact cause is not known.

Epidemiological studies of the metabolic syndrome conducted in the last fifty years have shown that in the countries in which the population is engaged in excessive eating and insufficient physical activity, the metabolic syndrome has reached almost epidemic proportions. About 15% of the population aged 40-75 years has a collection of diseases of the metabolic syndrome (Hanefeld and Kohler, 2002).

Numerous studies compared the prevalence of metabolic syndrome in some populations using different criteria. Using the criteria of the NCEP-ATP III, Canadian researchers found 33% prevalence of metabolic syndrome among persons aged between 40 and 60 years (Van den Hooven et al., 2006), while the survey conducted in 2008 in Japan under the same metabolic syndrome definition showed a prevalence of 8.1% for men and 9.9% for women in the total population (Lee et al., 2008).

The increase in the prevalence of metabolic syndrome is particularly evident in the United States (US), where in the periods from 1988 to 1994 and from 1999 to 2000, the age-standardized prevalence of the metabolic syndrome according to the NCEP-ATP III definition in the general population of people over 20 years of age, increased from 24.1% to 27.0% (Ford et al., 2004). The greatest increase in prevalence (23.5%) was recorded among women, while among men the prevalence of metabolic syndrome increased by 2.2% (Ford et al., 2004).

The prevalence of central type of obesity in the United States for the period from 1988 to 1994 amounted to 22.9%, while in the period from 1999 to 2000 increased to 30.5% (Ford et al., 2004).

Research of prevalence of metabolic syndrome among ethnic populations in the United States showed the lowest prevalence of metabolic syndrome in black men, slightly higher in whites, and highest in Hispanics (Ford et al., 2002).

It was observed that the prevalence of the metabolic syndrome is closely related to age. This is confirmed by a study conducted in Iran in 2003 when it was found that prevalence was <10% for men and women in the age group of 20-29 years, and that it was 38% for men and 67% for women in the age group of 60-69 years (Azizi et al., 2003).

In European countries the prevalence of the metabolic syndrome is also extensively studied. Although they used different definitions and research was conducted in the different sub-populations, the prevalence of the metabolic syndrome in the adult population ranged mostly between 15% (Hu et al., 2004) and 25% (Grundy, 2008).

In a study published in 2004, it was shown that the prevalence of the metabolic syndrome in France by NCEP ATP III was 23.0% for men and 16.9% for women aged 35 to 64 years old, while among people with advanced cardiovascular disease in the Netherlands it amounted to 46% (Gorter et al., 2004). According to the same definition of metabolic syndrome in the general population of Germany in the year 2007 the prevalence of metabolic syndrome was 23.5% for men and 17.6% for women (Assmann et al., 2007).

The prevalence of metabolic syndrome in 2005 in Italy was 15% for men, and 18% for women (Miccoli et al., 2005), while in Greece it totaled 24.5% (Athyros et al., 2005). Prevalence in Spain's population aged 35-64 years during 2006 amounted to 22.3% among men and 30.7% among women (Lorenzo et al., 2006).

The prevalence of metabolic syndrome in adults in Croatia in 2007 amounted to 8.8% in the group of 35-64 years of age (7.7% for men and 9.9% for women) and 19.6% in the age group over 65 years of age (15.2% for men and 22.5% for women), while in the total population the prevalence in males was 6.8%, and in females it was 10.3%. In this study, the metabolic syndrome was defined not according to internationally accepted conditions, but was based on persistently elevated waist circumference (> 102 cm for men and> 88 cm for women) and at least two of the following conditions: blood pressure ≥ 140/90 mmHg, a history of elevated cholesterol levels and a history of high blood sugar (Vuletic et al., 2007).

1.2. Diabetes and prediabetes

Diabetes mellitus encompasses a group of metabolic diseases characterized by hyperglycemia resulting from disorders of creation, secretion and/or insulin action (Anonymous, 2004).

Diagnostic criteria for the diagnosis of diabetes proposed by WHO (1998) are:
- glucose in whole blood glucose > 6.1 mmol/l or plasma glucose > 7.00 mmol/l (if the sample is from a vein or capillary) and
- glucose in whole blood 120 minutes after OGTT > 10.0 mmol/l (in case of the sample taken from a vein) or > 11.1 mmol/l (in case of the sample taken from capillaries), and plasma glucose > 11.1 mmol/l (in case of the sample taken from a vein) or > 12.2 mmol/l (in case of the sample taken from capillaries).

There are several types of diabetes. According to the etiology and clinical stages, most countries accept the classification of the American Diabetes Association (ADA) from 1997, which includes the following group of diseases:
- diabetes mellitus type 1;
   - Autoimmune form
   - Idiopathic form
- Diabetes mellitus type 2;
- Other specific types of diabetes due to other causes and
- Gestational diabetes form (Anonymous, 2004; Anonymous, 2007).

Type 1 diabetes is the result of autoimmune damage to the pancreatic β cells with subsequent insulin deficiency. Type 2 diabetes is caused by insulin resistance and insulin secretion disorders, and is often associated with obesity. Specific types of diabetes are classified as: genetic defects of β cell function, genetic defects of insulin action, diseases of the endocrine function of the pancreas, endocrinopathies, drug or chemically induced diabetes mellitus, rare forms of immune-mediated diseases and other genetic syndromes. Gestational diabetes is a type of disease which first manifests itself during pregnancy (Alberti, 2010).

In the foundation of all types of diabetes mellitus is a metabolic disorder caused by a number of factors. Chronic hyperglycemia characteristic of diabetes leads to disturbance of function and a damage of a number of organs and complications that are classified into microvascular complications and macrovascular complications. Most common microvascular complications are diabetic neuropathy, retinopathy and nephropathy, while most macrovascular complications include coronary heart disease, atherosclerosis and peripheral vascular disease (He et al., 2010).

The most common endocrine disease of the population of developed countries, according to estimates by the IDF, is the prevalence of diabetes mellitus, which in 2003 was 5.1% worldwide. In Europe it was 7.8% (Anonymous, 2003). In 2000, more than 151 million people suffered from diabetes, and it is estimated that by 2025 that number will grow to 324 million (Cheng, 2005).

The prevalence of diabetes varies widely in different populations and age groups. Also a clear difference in the prevalence of different types of diabetes mellitus has been established. Type 2 is the most common form and occurs in approximately 85-90% of all patients, while type 1 and other etiological types occur much less frequently. The prevalence of type 2 diabetes mellitus increases with age both in men and women (Balkau et al., 2004).

Prediabetes is a condition in which blood glucose levels are higher than normal but not high enough to be diagnosed as diabetes. This condition is sometimes called impaired fasting glucose (IFG) or impaired glucose tolerance (IGT), depending on the test used for diagnosis. Those disorders in glucose regulation are detected and differentiated by the OGTT measurement of fasting blood of plasma glucose levels 120 minutes after the glucose load (Peter and William, 2006).

Since 1979, the persons who on the OGTT have a score between normal values and values as in persons with severe disease (7.0 mmol/l to 11.0 mmol/l) are said to have IGT. A person with the values of fasting glucose of 5.6 mmol/l to 6.9 mmol/l has IFG (Anonymous, 2003).

The research showed that the measurement of glycated hemoglobin A1c (HbA1c), which determines the level of glucose in the blood for a period of the past three months, is easier and more reliable for determining the risk of diabetes mellitus type 2. However, the International Advisory Board does not recommend it for diagnosis, but only for disease control (Anonymous, 2003).

People with prediabetes are at increased risk of developing type 2 diabetes Studies show that most people with prediabetes develop diabetes over the next decade, if they do notlose 5-7% of their body weight. Insulin resistance and prediabetes usually have no symptoms. People can have either one or both conditions for several years without noticing it (Santaguida et al., 2005). Long-term hyperglycaemia is associated with complications in the form of organ damage and dysfunction of various organs, especially the eyes, kidneys, nerves, and blood vessels (Anonymous, 2004).

1.3. Neuropathy in metabolic syndrome

Neuropathy is a clinical condition of a minor or severe illness of the affected nerve. Polyneuropathy usually refers to the involvement of more peripheral nerves, with mostly symmetrical distribution. Diabetic neuropathy is the most common complication of diabetes and also the most common disease of the peripheral nerves in the developed countries (Kostic et al., 2009).

The prevalence of polyneuropathy in time of detection of diabetes mellitus was 7.5%, and 25 years after it rises to 50% (Shaw et al., 2003). The prevalence of symptomatic forms (painful polyneuropathy) is about 13%, and it develops in both type-1 and in the type-2 diabetes in (Pirart, 1978).

Diabetic neuropathy includes a number of different, well-defined types of damage to the nervous system, whose diversity suggests several possible pathophysiological mechanisms. The factors that lead to polyneuropathy in patients with diabetes mellitus still have not been fully explained, but it is generally accepted that it is a combination of multiple causal factors such as metabolic and hemodynamic changes, lack of neurotrophic factors, and autoimmunity (Yasuda et al., 2003 ; He et al., 2004; Witzke and Vinik, 2005; Greene et al., 1999). To distinguish certain forms of diabetic neuropathy it is necessary to assess symptoms and clinical signs, and to conduct neurophysiological testing.

Clinical classification of diabetic neuropathy, modified according to Dyck (Dyck and Taylor, 1999):

1. Diabetic polyneuropathy
2. Focal and multifocal neuropathies
    • Proximal diabetic neuropathy
    • Compression neuropathy
    • Neuropathies of brain nerves
    • Truncal radiculoneuropathies

3. Neuropathy of the autonomic nervous system

Of these the most common types (found in 72% of patients), distal polyneuropathy, in 12% of cases is the syndrome of carpal tunnel, other mononeuropathies are represented in 6% of cases, while other neuropathies occurred in 10% of these patients. Approximately 10% of patients with diabetes mellitus have a different form of neuropathy that is not caused by diabetes alone (Dyck and Melton, 1999).

Metabolic syndrome is much more common in patients with neuropathy, whether they have normal glucose regulation or impaired glucose tolerance (Smith and Singleton, 2008).

Metabolic syndrome may be responsible for the symptoms of nerve compression in the anatomical constrictions such as carpal and Gyon channel in the wrist or hypothenar or channel ulnar nerve at the elbow. Peripheral nerve in patients with diabetes mellitus is particularly sensitive to pressure, stretching or repeated mechanical trauma. It is assumed that this is a disorder in the recovery of nerves in places that are otherwise exposed to damage (Barada et al., 2000; Moughtaderi and Ghafarpoor, 2009). It has been shown also that oxidative stress (an imbalance in production of reactive species of oxygen and the ability of tissue cells to detoxify free radicals during the metabolic activity) contribute to the pathology of neural and vascular dysfunction in diabetes (Pop-Busua et al., 2006).

Electroneurography of peripheral nerves through the use of surface stimulation and registration electrodes represents the most sensitive and the most easily reproducible method of all the neurophysiological tests for neuropathy (Dyck et al., 1997; Arezzo, 1999; Behsa et al., 1977; Daub, 1980; Valensi and Atal, 1993). This method analyzes the function of myelinated neurons. The places of electrical stimulation of certain nerves and registration of evoked responses are determined by standard procedure (Anonymous, 1995). Timings and forms of evoked response, and motor and sensory nerve conduction velocities are indicators of myelin sheath condition. Demyelination (partial or diffuse) will reduce nerve conduction velocity. Lower amplitude of potential is proportional to the number of fibers in the conduction. The lower potential amplitude indicates damage (degeneration) of axons. In diabetes mellitus or in the metabolic syndrome, polyneuropathic changes lead to significantly damaged sensory nerve fibers, which is why the first sign of polyneuropathy can be paresthesia (Said et al., 1983).

Dominant changes in patients with no subjective signs of polyneuropathy were demyelination and remyelination, while patients with severe signs of polyneuropathy show combined demyelination and remyelination damage with signs of axonal degeneration (Thomas and Tomlinson, 1993). In the painful diabetic polyneuropathy, loss of thin myelinated fibers prevails, together with degeneration and regeneration of non-myelinated axons (Said et al., 1983; Brown et al., 1976).

It is known that polyneuropathy equally affects both sexes, and that it is more common in the elderly and in a small percentage in children with diabetes (about 2%). However, there is a lot of unknowns about the nature of origin, development in the various time stages and consequences of neuropathy in metabolic syndrome on the functioning of the body and quality of life of patients with this disease.

1.4. Research goals

1. Identify electroneurographic parameters for ulnar and median nerves in patients with metabolic syndrome who have normal glucoregulation, prediabetes and diabetes duration of up to five years.

2. To determine whether the disorders of neurophysiological parameters are associated with a pronounced imbalance in glucoregulation.

1.5. Hypotheses

Working hypotheses

1. Neurophysiological parameters in patients with the metabolic syndrome and prediabetes or diabetes mellitus with duration of up to five years have been changed compared to the same parameters of subjects with metabolic syndrome and normal glucoregulation.

2. Changes in neurophysiological parameters were more pronounced in patients with a greater imbalance in glucoregulation.

Null hypothesis

1. Neurophysiological parameters in patients with metabolic syndrome and prediabetes or diabetes mellitus with duration of up to five years have not been changed when compared to the same parameters of subjects with metabolic syndrome and normal glucoregulation.
2. Changes in neurophysiological parameters are not more pronounced in patients with a greater imbalance in glucoregulation.

2. Patients and Methods

2.1. Patients

The study was retrospective-prospective and included all patients with metabolic syndrome registered in twelve teams of family medicine of the Health Center and Polyclinic "Dr Mustafa Šehović" in Tuzla. The study included subjects of both genders and of all age groups. The diagnosis of metabolic syndrome was based on lab tests and anthropometric measurements, and taking into account the criteria of the NCEP-ATP III for the diagnosis of metabolic syndrome (Anonymous, 2001). The studies excluded subjects with diabetes mellitus type 1, respondents who amputated one or both upper limbs, then those who have had surgery or injury of deeper tissues and/or who have had a tumor process localized in the areas of proliferation of nerves to be tested. Furthermore, respondents who have had uremia, hereditary neuropathy or autoimmune disease with neuropathic symptoms.

In the research project the target group was defined to have 150 patients. The first patient selection was made based on the data in the medical records: data on diabetes mellitus, result of anthropometric measurements (waist), values of blood pressure and laboratory analyses (triglycerides and high-density lipoprotein). For differentiation of the degree of disorder in glukoregulation, OGTT was used (120 minutes after the load). Based on these results, respondents were divided into three equal groups: The first group consisted of 50 respondents with metabolic syndrome and normal glukoregulation, of which 14 were male. The average age of respondents was 52.6 (38-65) ± 3.3 years. The average value of the blood sugar glucose measured was 5.1 (4-5,5) ± 0.4 mmol/l. The average value of blood sugar two hours after the OGTT was 4.5 (2.2 to 6.1) ± 0.9mmol/l. The average waist circumference was 104 (88 to 148) ± 11.2 cm. The average value of systolic blood pressure was 134 (110-160) ± 11mmHg, and diastolic 88.4 (70-100) ± 6.7 mmHg. The average value of high

19

density lipoprotein amounted to 1.2 (0.8-1.9) ± 0.2 mmol/l. The average triglyceride value was 2.8 (0.9 to 12.3) ± 1,9 mmol/l.

The second group consisted of 50 patients who as part of the metabolic syndrome had prediabetes, of which 25 were male. The average age of respondents was 54.1 (39-67) ± 7god. The average measured value of fasting blood sugar glucose was 6.4 (5.7 to 7.6) ± 0.5 mmol/l. The average value of blood glucose after OGTT was 5.6 (2.7 to 9.8) ± 1.7 mmol/l. The average waist circumference amounted to 104.7 (86-140) ± 11cm. The average value of systolic blood pressure was 133.5 (100-160) ± 10.9 mmHg and of diastolic blood pressure was 89.6 (60-180) ± 15.2 mmHg. The average value of high density lipoprotein amounted to 1.2 (0.7 to 1.7) ± 0.2 mmol/l. The average triglyceride value was 2.5 (0.9 to 8.2) ± 1.3mmol/l.

The third group consisted of 50 patients who as part of the metabolic syndrome had type 2 diabetes mellitus for up to five years. Of those 50 patients, 19 were male. The average age of respondents was 61 (38-78) ± 9.7 years of age. The average value of the measured fasting blood sugar was 8.3 (5.3 to 12.3) ± 1.5 mmol/l. The average value of blood glucose after OGTT was 11.7 (5.4 to 18.2) ± 2.7 mmol/l. The average waist size was 107 (85-142) ± 13.5cm. The average value of systolic blood pressure was 142.3 (100-200) ± 21.4 mmHg and the average value of the diastolic blood pressure was 87.2 (70-120) ± 11.1 mmHg. The average value of high density lipoprotein was 1.1 (0.5 to 2.4) ± 0.4 mmol/l. The average triglyceride value was 3.1 (0.6 to 12.2) ± 1.9mmol/l.

After collecting these data, the following electroneurographic parameters were measured in respondents: sensory conductive velocity (SCV), amplitude of sensory nerve action potential (SNAP), motor conductive velocity (MCV), terminal motor latency (TML) and complexes of muscular action potentials after distal stimulation

(CMAP-I) and after proximal stimulation (CMAP-II), in median and ulnar nerves of both arms.

The study was approved by the Ethics Committee of the Health Center Tuzla. The respondents gave their written consent to be included in the study. The study was stopped when the planned sample was collected.

2.2. Methods

All subjects were tested electroneurographically. Electroneurographic testing of subjects was conducted at room temperature and the "physiological" temperature of the skin in a horizontal position. To measure neurographic parameters electroneurographic instrument Medelec Synergy was used (EMG and EP Systems - OXFORD INSTRUMENTS 2004). Superficial stimulating and registration bipolar (aka. Large Touchproof) electrodes were utilized.

Measurement of MCS in the left and right median nerve was carried out by stimulating the nerves in the wrist and elbow and by registration in musculus abductor pollicis brevis. SCV in the left and right median nerve was measured by stimulating nerves in the wrist and registration on the junction of the first and second phalanx of the second finger. MCS of the left and right ulnar nerve was measured by stimulating nerves at the wrist and elbow and registration in musculus abductor digiti minimi. SCV of the left and right ulnar nerves was measured by stimulating nerves at the wrist and registration on the junction of the first and second phalanx of the fifth finger.

In electroneurographic processing the following were analyzed: sensory conduction velocity (SCV) in the hand and the highest amplitude of SNAP, and motor conduction velocity (MCV) in the forearm and CMAP area. Speeds are measured in meters per second (m/s). Stimulation in determining motor and sensory responses was performed up to the top of the CMAP and SNAP amplitudes. In cases where a sensory response was not received, the rate of implementation was recorded as 0 m/s.

2.3. Statistical Analysis

Values measured during the study are shown in the tables. For the processing of data relating to the grouping of patients as the measure of central tendency arithmetic mean was used, and as a measure of dispersion, the minimum and maximum values and standard deviations were used. To process the data obtained by measurements, as a measure of the central tendency the median was used, and as a measure of dispersion of the 25th and 75th percentile and the minimum and maximum value were used (Fazlović, 2006). To test the hypothesis, because of inhomogeneities of variance, the nonparametric Mann-Whitney U-test was employed to test the hypothesis bi-directionally (Petz, 1997). For all the statistical tests the level of significance of 5% was considered statistically significant. All statistical analysis was done in Microsoft Office Excel 2007 and Arcus Quickstat Biomedical program for statistical data processing.

3. Results

3.1. The Results of Measurement of Electroneurographical Parameters

Parameters of motor and sensory neurographic analysis of median and ulnar nerves in 50 patients with metabolic syndrome and normal glucoregulation are shown in the following tables (tables 1 and 2).

Table 1. Parameters of sensory neurographic analysis of median and ulnaris nerves in 50 patients with the metabolic syndrome and normal glucoregulation

Parameter	Nerve	Median	Percentile (25-75)	Min.	Max.
Conduction velocity (m/s)	n.medianus sin.	50.0	43.7 - 54.8	0.0	62.2
	n.medianus dex.	48.9	43.7 - 52.6	0.0	60.0
	n.ulnaris sin.	48.2	46.3 - 51.0	36.2	58.5
	n.ulnaris dex.	49.1	45.9 - 52.1	36.4	59.5
SNAP Amplitude (µV)	n.medianus sin.	17.3	10.0 - 23.1	0.0	32.7
	n.medianus dex.	14.8	9.6 - 19.9	0.0	26.4
	n.ulnaris sin.	20.2	11.7 - 27.4	5.2	51.1
	n.ulnaris dex.	18.2	12.6 - 28.6	2.3	52.3

Min.- minimum; Max.- maximum; sin.- left (lat. *sinister*); dex.- right (lat. *dexter*); SNAP- sensory nerve action potential

In this group in two respondents it was not possible to cause SNAP in the left median nerve, and in three patients it was not possible to do it in the right median nerve, which is why, as the table above shows, the minimum value of conduction velocity and amplitude of SNAP is marked as 0 m/s or 0 µV.

Table 2. Parameters of motor neurographic analysis of the median and ulnaris nerves in 50 patients with the metabolic syndrome and normal glucoregulation

Parameter	Nerve	Median	Percentile (25-75)	Min.	Max.
Conduction velocity (m/s)	n. medianus sin.	56.0	54.0 - 59.5	44.8	69.7
	n. medianus dex.	55.9	53.2 - 59.2	47.5	66.6
	n. ulnaris sin.	53.5	51.0 - 55.5	44.8	64.9
	n. ulnaris dex.	54.1	51.0 - 56.4	47.1	67.6
Terminal latency (ms)	n. medianus sin.	3.4	3.1 - 3.8	1.8	5.5
	n. medianus dex.	3.6	3.1 - 3.9	2.6	9.5
	n. ulnaris sin.	2.8	2.5 - 3.0	2.1	3.9
	n. ulnaris dex.	3.0	2.5 - 3.2	1.9	4.0
CMAP-I surface (mVms)	n. medianus sin.	20.6	14.8 - 31.0	6.0	42.3
	n. medianus dex.	24.3	19.5 - 32.1	6.9	44.9
	n. ulnaris sin.	18.5	13.7 - 22.3	5.5	37.1
	n. ulnaris dex.	15.4	11.8 - 20.9	3.6	31.0
CMAP-II surface (mVms)	n. medianus sin.	19.8	13.8 - 26.7	6.5	41.0
	n. medianus dex.	21.9	17.8 - 28.2	6.9	42.9
	n. ulnaris sin.	16.3	11.2 - 21.0	5.2	35.7
	n. ulnaris dex.	14.7	11.2 - 18.7	3.7	28.4

Min.- minimum; Max.- maximum; sin.- left (lat. *sinister*); dex.- right (lat. *dexter*); CMAP-I – muscular action potential complex following distal stimulation; CMAP-II - muscular action potential complex following proximal stimulation.

Parameters of motor and sensory neurographic analysis of median and ulnar nerves in 50 patients who had both the metabolic syndrome and prediabetes, are shown in the following tables (tables 3 and 4).

Table 3. Parameters of sensory neurographic analysis of median and ulnar nerves in 50 patients who had prediabetes as part of their metabolic syndrome

Parameter	Nerve	Median	Percentile (25 -75)	Min.	Max.
Conduction velocity (m/s)	n.medianus sin.	47.9	44.8 - 50.8	27.5	57.3
	n.medianus dex.	46.9	43.1 - 49.4	29.5	58.9
	n.ulnaris sin.	47.1	44.6 - 49.0	19.8	55.0
	n.ulnaris dex.	47.0	44.0 - 49.1	35.3	55.6
SNAP amplitude (μV)	n.medianus sin.	12.0	9.0 - 16.7	2.7	31.3
	n.medianus dex.	10.6	8.1 - 16.7	4.7	49.7
	n.ulnaris sin.	14.4	10.4 - 18.1	5.9	31.0
	n.ulnaris dex.	15.7	10.7 - 20.0	4.2	39.0

Min.- minimum; Max.- maximum; sin.- left (lat. *sinister*); dex.- right (lat. *dexter*); SNAP- sensory nerve action potential

In all the patients in this group it was possible to cause SNAP. However, it can be seen that in all tested nerves, the sensory conducting velocity is lower, and that the median values of SNAP amplitudes are lower than in the first group (the group with the subjects with metabolic syndrome and normal glucoregulation).

The differences in terms of moving towards the neuropathic pattern were recorded in nearly all motor components of electroneurographic analysis (motor velocity conducting, terminal latency, CMAP-I and CMAP-II surface) in this group than in the group of subjects with the metabolic syndrome and normal glucoregulation.

Table 4. Parameters of motor neurographic analysis of median and ulnar nerves in 50 respondents who, as part of the metabolic syndrome, had prediabetes

Parameter	Nerve	Median	Percentile (25-75)	Min.	Max.
Conduction velocity (m/s)	n. medianus sin.	55.7	51.7 - 59.0	44.0	63.5
	n. medianus dex.	54.6	52.5 - 56.6	34.0	65.0
	n. ulnaris sin.	51.4	48.7 – 53.5	32.4	61.1
	n. ulnaris dex.	52.8	50.4 - 55.7	46.8	63.4
Terminal latency (ms)	n. medianus sin.	3.6	3.4 - 3.9	2.6	4.9
	n. medianus dex.	3.5	3.3 - 3.9	2.3	5.2
	n. ulnaris sin.	3.0	2.7 - 3.1	2.0	3.9
	n. ulnaris dex.	3.1	2.7 - 3.3	1.9	4.1
CMAP-I surface (mVms)	n. medianus sin.	22.3	17.3 - 26.2	10.5	43.9
	n. medianus dex.	19.9	15.8 - 26.7	6.6	47.6
	n. ulnaris sin.	15.9	12.6 - 20.7	4.1	42.6
	n. ulnaris dex.	17.3	11.2 - 20.5	4.5	49.2
CMAP-II surface (mVms)	n. medianus sin.	19.5	15.6 - 24.1	6.3	39.4
	n. medianus dex.	17.1	13.4 - 24.9	3.7	46.8
	n. ulnaris sin.	14.1	9.9 - 18.3	3.8	36.6
	n. ulnaris dex.	15.2	10.2 - 19.0	4.0	46.8

Min.- minimum; Max.- maximum; sin.- left (lat. *sinister*); dex.- right (lat. *dexter*); CMAP-I – muscular action potential following distal stimulation; CMAP-II – muscular action potential following proximal stimulation

Parameters of motor and sensory neurographic analysis of median and ulnar nerves in 50 respondents who, as part of the metabolic syndrome, had diabetes for up to five years, are shown in the following tables (tables 5 and 6).

Table 5. Parameters of sensory neurographic analysis of median and ulnar nerves in 50 respondents who, as part of the metabolic syndrome, had diabetes for up to five years

Parameter	Nerve	Median	Percentile (25 - 75)	Min.	Max.
Conduction velocity (m/s)	n.medianus sin.	44.8	38.7 – 50.6	0.0	61.5
	n.medianus dex.	43.2	38.7 - 49.7	0.0	57.4
	n.ulnaris sin.	44.2	41.2 - 48.2	0.0	56.0
	n.ulnaris dex.	44.8	41.0 - 48.7	0.0	55.3
SNAP Amplitude (µV)	n.medianus sin.	9.1	5.3 - 13.5	0.0	39.0
	n.medianus dex.	7.6	4.0 - 12.0	0.0	24.3
	n.ulnaris sin.	9.6	6.6 - 15.5	0.0	34.5
	n.ulnaris dex.	10.3	7.9 - 15.3	0.0	29.4

Min.- minimum; Max.- maximum; sin.- sinister (lat. left); dex.- dexter (lat. right); SNAP- sensory nerve action potential

In this group, in four respondents it was not possible to cause SNAP in the left median nerve, and in two cases it was not possible to do it in the left ulnar nerve. In six respondents SNAP could not be caused in the right median nerve, and in one case this was not possible in the right ulnar nerve. The median rate of sensory conducting and SNAP amplitudes are lower than in the first two groups of patients (subjects with normal glucoregulation and subjects with prediabetes). The differences in terms of moving towards a more pronounced neuropathic pattern were recorded in nearly all motor components of electroneurographic analysis of these nerves.

Table 6. Parameters of motor neurographic analysis of median and ulnar nerves in 50 respondents who had diabetes for up to five years, as part of their metabolic syndrome

Parameter	Nerve	Median	Percentile (25-75)	Min.	Max.
Conduction velocity (m/s)	n. medianus sin.	53.5	50.2 - 56.8	40.9	61.3
	n. medianus dex.	53.0	50.0 - 56.8	29.5	60.8
	n. ulnaris sin.	49.5	46.1 - 51.7	23.7	68.4
	n. ulnaris dex.	49.7	45.3 - 52.6	31.8	62.2
Terminal latency (ms)	n. medianus sin.	3.9	3.4 - 4.2	2.8	6.9
	n. medianus dex.	3.9	3.5 - 4.1	2.9	8.8
	n. ulnaris sin.	3.1	2.8 - 3.3	2.0	5.4
	n. ulnaris dex.	3.0	2.6 - 3.5	2.0	7.3
CMAP-I surface (mVms)	n. medianus sin.	18.7	14.3 - 25.3	2.6	41.2
	n. medianus dex.	20.4	16.3 - 27.3	6.0	40.7
	n. ulnaris sin.	15.1	12.3 - 20.6	2.6	31.7
	n. ulnaris dex.	12.4	9.7 - 16.8	4.7	26.8
CMAP-II surface (mVms)	n. medianus sin.	17.3	11.9 - 23.8	1.9	38.7
	n. medianus dex.	19.1	14.9 - 25.8	5.1	37.0
	n. ulnaris sin.	14.7	11.0 - 19.1	1.9	30.1
	n. ulnaris dex.	12.0	8.4 - 15.6	2.8	24.8

Min.- minimum; Max.- maximum; sin.- left (lat. *sinister*); dex.- right (lat. *dexter*); CMAP I – muscular action potential complex following distal stimulation; CMAP II - muscular action potential complex following proximal stimulation.

3.2. Significance of differences in electroneurographical parameters

Testing of the parameters of sensory and motor neurographic analysis of median and ulnar nerves in the first group of 50 patients with the metabolic syndrome and normal glucoregulation, and the second group of 50 patients who had prediabetes as part of their metabolic syndrome, has produced a significantly lower SNAP amplitude in the left median nerve, a significantly lower conducting velocity and SNAP amplitude for the left ulnar nerve, and significantly lower rate of sensory conducting in the right ulnar nerve in the second group. As for the motor components, the second group had significantly lower values of CMAP-I and CMAP-II surface in the right median nerve, as well as terminal motor latency values for the left ulnar nerve (tables 7 and 8).

Table 7. The significance of differences in the parameters of sensory neurographic analysis of median and ulnar nerves in 50 patients with the metabolic syndrome and normal glucoregulation, and 50 patients with prediabetes as part of their metabolic syndrome

Nerve	Parameter	p...
n.medianus sin.	Velocity	0.1844
	SNAP amplitude	0.0376
n. medianus dex.	Velocity	0.2303
	SNAP amplitude	0.1733
n.ulnaris sin.	Velocity	0.0448
	Amplituda SNAP	0.0062
n.ulnaris dex.	Brzina	0.0225
	SNAP amplitude	0.0787

p ...- the possibility of random differences in the two-sided hypotheses; sin.- left (lat. *sinister*); dex.- right (lat. *dexter*); SNAP- sensory nerve action potential.

Table 8. The significance of differences in the parameters of the motor neurographic analysis of median and ulnar nerves in 50 patients with the metabolic syndrome and normal glucoregulation, and 50 patients who had prediabetes as part of their metabolic syndrome

Nerve	Parameter	p...
n.medianus sin.	Conduction velocity	0.2524
	Terminal latency	0.0929
	CMAP-I surface	0.5719
	CMAP-II surface	0.9862
n. medianus dex.	Conduction velocity	0.0829
	Terminal latency	0.6366
	CMAP-I surface	0.0301
	CMAP-II surface	0.0315
n.ulnaris sin.	Conduction velocity	0.0060
	Terminal latency	0.0431
	CMAP-I surface	0.1506
	CMAP-II surface	0.1526
n. ulnaris dex.	Conduction velocity	0.1311
	Terminal latency	0.5952
	CMAP-I surface	0.8254
	CMAP-II surface	0.8415

p ...- possibility of random differences of two-sided hypotheses; sin.- left; dex.- right; CMAP-I - compound muscle action potential following distal stimulation; CMAP-II - compound muscle action potential following proximal stimulation.

Testing of the parameters of sensory and motor neurographic analysis of median and ulnar nerves in the second group of 50 patients, who, as part of their metabolic syndrome, had prediabetes, and the third group of 50 patients, who had diabetes for up to five years as part of their metabolic syndrome. Thus, in the third group of patients (metabolic syndrome and diabetes lasting up to five years) significantly lower values were found in all sensory parameters of the left ulnar nerve, SNAP amplitudes of both median nerves and the right ulnar nerve; the value of terminal motor latencies of the right median nerve, the motor conduction velocity of the left ulnar nerve, and motor conduction velocity, CMAP-I and II on the surfaces of the right ulnar nerve (tables 9 and 10).

Table 9. The significance of differences in the parameters of sensory neurographic analysis of median and ulnar nerves in 50 respondents who had prediabetes as part of their metabolic syndrome, and 50 respondents who had diabetes for up to five years as part of their metabolic syndrome

Nerve	Parameter	p...
n.medianus sin	Velocity	0.0580
	SNAP amplitude	0.0082
n. medianus dex.	Velocity	0.0598
	SNAP amplitude	0.0008
n.ulnaris sin.	Velocity	0.0326
	SNAP amplitude	0.0023
n.ulnaris dex.	Velocity	0.1184
	SNAP amplitude	0.0027

p ...- possibility of random differences in the two-sided hypothesis; sin.- left (lat. *sinister*); dex.- right (lat. *dexter*); SNAP- sensory nerve action potential

Table 10. The significance of the differences in the parameters of the motor neurographic analysis of median and ulnar nerves in 50 respondents who had prediabetes as part of their metabolic syndrome, and in 50 respondents who had diabetes for up to five years as part of their metabolic syndrome

Nerve	Parameter	p...
n.medianus sin.	Conduction velocity	0.0703
	Terminal latency	0.1407
	CMAP-I surface	0.2046
	CMAP-II surface	0.1392
n. medianus dex.	Conduction velocity	0.0867
	Terminal latency	0.0256
	CMAP-I surface	0.7355
	CMAP-II surface	0.3984
n.ulnaris sin.	Conduction velocity	0.0185
	Terminal latency	0.1470
	CMAP-I surface	0.9615
	CMAP-II surface	0.8822
n.ulnaris dex.	Conduction velocity	0.0002
	Terminal latency	0.5347
	CMAP-I surface	0.0253
	CMAP-II surface	0.0151

p ...- possibility of random differences in the two-sided hypothesis; sin.- left (lat. *sinister*); dex.- right (lat. *dexter*); CMAP-I - compound muscle action potential following distal stimulation; CMAP -II - compound muscle action potential following proximal stimulation.

Testing of the differences in parameters of sensory and motor neurographic analysis of median and ulnar nerves in the first group of 50 patients with the metabolic syndrome and normal glucoregulation, and the third group of 50 patients who had diabetes for up to five years as part of their metabolic syndrome. Thus, in the third group of patients (metabolic syndrome and diabetes duration of up to five years), significantly lower values were found in all sensory parameters of both nerves: for the motor conductivity velocity of ulnar nerves, for the terminal motor latency conductivity of both median nerves and the left ulnar nerve, for the the CMAP-I surface of each nerve of the right hand and CMAP-II of right ulnar nerves (tables 11 and 12).

Table 11. The significance of differences in the parameters of sensory neurographical analysis of median and ulnar nerves in 50 patients with metabolic syndrome and normal glucoregulations, and 50 patients who had diabetes for up to five years, as part of their metabolic syndrome

Nerve	Parameter	p…
n.medianus sin.	Velocity	0.0099
	SNAP Amplitude	p<0.0001
n. medianus dex.	Velocity	0.0107
	SNAP Amplitude	p<0.0001
n.ulnaris sin.	Velocity	0.0005
	SNAP Amplitude	p<0.0001
n.ulnaris dex.	Velocity	0.0008
	SNAP Amplitude	p<0.0001

p …- possibility of random differences in the two-sided hypothesis; sin.- left (lat. *sinister*); dex.- right (lat. *dexter*); SNAP- sensory nerve action potential

Table 12. The significance of the differences in the parameters of the motor neurographical analysis of the median and ulnar nerves in 50 patients with metabolic syndrome and normal glucoregulation and 50 patients who had diabetes for up to five years as part of their metabolic syndrome

Nerve	Parameter	p...
n.medianus sin.	Conduction velocity	0.0030
	Terminal latency	0.0130
	CMAP-I surface	0.4279
	CMAP-II surface	0.1458
n. medianus dex.	Conduction velocity	0.0012
	Terminal latency	0.0112
	CMAP-I surface	0.0437
	CMAP-II surface	0.1067
n.ulnaris sin.	Conduction velocity	$p<0.0001$
	Terminal latency	0.0023
	CMAP-I surface	0.1184
	CMAP-II surface	0.2022
n. ulnaris dex.	Conduction velocity	$p<0.0001$
	Terminal latency	0.3482
	CMAP-I surface	0.0358
	CMAP-II surface	0.0184

p ...- possibility of random differences in the two-sided hypothesis; sin.- left (lat. *sinister*); dex.- right (lat. *dexter*); CMAP-I - compound muscle action potential following distal stimulation; CMAP -II - compound muscle action potential following proximal stimulation.

4. Discussion

Although not immediately recognizable during the classical neurological examination, neuropathies are common disorders that accompany metabolic syndrome. Timely insight into these changes may determine further therapeutic strategy. Its aim should be to prevent further progression of the syndrome and its potential destructive effects on the peripheral nerves, which in turn can impair the function and therefore adversely affect the very quality of life of patients with this syndrome.

This study suggests that the metabolic syndrome is more common in women. Specifically, in a continuous sample of 150 subjects with metabolic syndrome nearly 2/3 (61.4%) were female, and in a little more than 1/3 (38.6%) of cases these were men. Similar data have been reported in most of the Mediterranean countries (Spain, Italy and Croatia) (Lorenzo et al., 2006; Micolli et al., 2005; Vuletic et al., 2007). The studies that are related to the incidence of metabolic syndrome in Germany and France have shown that it is more common among males (Gorter et al., 2004; Assmann et al., 2007).

It is noted also that the disorder in glucoregulation in people with the metabolic syndrome is positively correlated with age. The average age of patients in the group with normal glucoregulation was 52 years; in the group of subjects with prediabetes it was 54, and in the group of patients with diabetes lasting for up to five years, it was 61 years of age. This connection is confirmed by studies conducted by Bakau et al. (2004).

This study further showed that waist circumference in patients with metabolic syndrome positively correlates with the degree of disorder in glucoregulation, where a more pronounced increase in the values of waist circumference is recorded in subjects with evident diabetes. Furthermore, subjects with metabolic syndrome and a higher degree of disorder in glucoregulation (diabetes lasting for up to five years) had lower values of high-density lipoprotein, and higher values of triglycerides and systolic blood pressure when compared to subjects with normal glucoregulation or prediabetes. This could be explained by close relatedness of the components of the metabolic syndrome and that they ultimately both cause and affect each other, which is confirmed by the pathophysiological mechanisms of the metabolic syndrome and its impact on the functioning of the organism as a whole.

4.1. Electroneurographic Parameters in Patients with the Metabolic Syndrome and Normal lucoregulation

Results of this study showed that in the group of patients with the metabolic syndrome and normal glucoregulation, SNAP could not be caused in the left median nerve in two cases, and in the right median nerve in three cases. Therefore, the velocity of sensory conductivity could not be measured in those nerves. This suggests that the neuropathic changes were present in this group of patients also.

In the literature, there is little data on the frequency of neuropathy as part of the metabolic syndrome without diabetes mellitus. Smith et al. (2008), published the results of their research: The incidence of neuropathy in people with the meatbolic syndrome and normal glucoregulation is greater than the rate in the general population. The same survey showed a higher prevalence of dyslipidemia in patients with neuropathy than in patients without neuropathy.

Our research showed that the largest number of changed parameters in the group of patients with the metabolic syndrome and normal glucoregulation was related to sensory components of neurographical analysis. This indicates a pronounced vulnerability of sensory fibers in peripheral nerves. The research conducted by Said et al. (1983) showed that the paresthesia as a sign of damage to the sensory nerve function is identified as the first symptom of peripheral polyneuropathy.

Furthermore, it was shown that in the group of patients with the metabolic syndrome and normal glucoregulation, the most vulnerable was the right median nerve. This can be explained by the fact that the peripheral nerves that are located in anatomic constrictions (carpal tunnel, Guyon's canal or cubital ulnar nerve at the elbow) are constantly under pressure, stretching or repeated mechanical trauma. In patients with the metabolic syndrome nerves are more sensitive and slower to recover from the consequences of damage (Barada et al., 2000; Moughtaderi and Ghafarpoor, 2009). It is assumed that the most likely cause of the said slow recovery is the slower axonal transport, which maintains the nerve metabolism and helps in its recovery. Furthermore, it is commonly known that the majority of the population is right-handed, and thus it is assumed that in the study group, that ratio is approximately the same. Taking all this into consideration, it can be assumed that the right-handed subjects with metabolic syndrome have a higher chance that the carpal tunnel compressed right median and damages the nerve and thus leads to changes in sensory components of the electroneurographic analysis.

The inability to cause SNAP in the median nerve in this group of patients indicates the presence of carpal tunnel syndrome. Research by Onder et al. (2012) found that of 150 patients with the carpal tunnel syndrome, 73.5% of them have had the metabolic syndrome. Furthermore, subjects with the metabolic syndrome had significantly more difficult forms of carpal tunnel syndrome as compared to patients without the metabolic syndrome.

4.2. Electroneurographic parameters in patients who had prediabetes as part of their metabolic syndrome

Results of this study showed that a greater number of electroneurographical parameters in the group of patients that had the metabolic syndrome with prediabetes, is in a statistically significant measure changed towards a neuropathic pattern, when compared to the same parameters of patients with the metabolic syndrome and normal glucoregulation.

In a study conducted by Papanas et al. (2011) it has been shown that between 25% and 62% of patients with idiopathic peripheral neuropathy have prediabetes. Another study conducted by the same researchers found that the incidence of neuropathy in a group of subjects with prediabetes is between the frequency of neuropathy in a group of patients with overt diabetes mellitus and the incidence in the group of patients with normal glucoregulation, and that among them there was a generally milder form of neuropathy which mainly affected small fibers responsible for sensory functions (Papanas et al., 2012).

In a recently published study it is stated that peripheral neuropathy can develop in patients with prediabetes and metabolic syndrome before they manifest diabetes mellitus, and that it is still not known which factor contributes more to nerve damage (insulin intolerance, hypertriglyceridemia and/or increased concentration of free fatty acids) (Lupachyk et al., 2012).

Based on the aforementioned, we believe that further research is needed to better define the association between the glucoregulation, the metabolic syndrome and neuropathy. It is necessary to expand on pathophysiological basis for their creation and development. It is necessary, in accordance with the results of research, to take appropriate measures and develop strategies for the diagnosis and therapeutic action aimed at the patients with such diseases. A better understanding of the mechanisms that lead to the metabolic syndrome, as well as the consequences which it brings, will be useful in the prevention and treatment of patients with this disease.

4.3. Electroneurographic parameters in patients with the metabolic syndrome with diabetes lasting for up to five years

The results of this study have showed that almost all values of the electroneurographical parameters on the median and ulnar nerves, in the group of patients with both the metabolic syndrome and diabetes lasting for up to five years, are statistically significantly changed towards the neuropathic pattern in relation to the value of the same parameter in the group of patients with the metabolic syndrome and normal glucoregulation.

There is an enormous number of published studies that confirm the adverse impact of diabetes mellitus on the occurrence and development of neuropathy. Shaw et al. (2003) published the results of a study that says that the incidence of diabetic neuropathy increases with age, duration of diabetes and bad glycemic control, and this is confirmed by our observations.

This research has shown that in accordance with the development of the neuropathic pattern within the metabolic syndrome, in most cases the expected changes of individual neurophysiological parameters do happen.

The values of terminal motor latencies for individual nerves are longer in the group of patients who had prediabetes as part of their metabolic syndrome, than in the group of subjects with normal glucoregulation. However, they are the longest in the group of patients with diabetes lasting for up to five years.

In accordance with the metabolic changes imposed by the motor nerve conduction, it is found that the motor nerve conduction velocity in the median and ulnar nerves is lower in the group of respondents that had prediabetes as a part of their metabolic syndrome, than in the group of respondents with normal glucoregulation, and that the lowest velocities were found in the group of subjects with diabetes lastign for up to five years. Therefore, the deceleration was more pronounced with a more pronounced imbalance in glucoregulation.

Also, research has shown that the differences are more evident when it comes to comparison in conduction velocity in the ulnar nerves. This can be explained with the anatomical position of the ulnar nerves in the elbow, which are exposed to stretching, pressure and other forms of damage daily.

Values of CMAP areas were reduced with the development of the neuropathic sample, so that the maximum areas were present in the group of subjects with the metabolic syndrome and normal glucoregulation; they were lower in the group of subjects that had the metabolic syndrome with prediabetes; finally they were the lowest in the group of respondents with the metabolic syndrome and diabetes lasting for up to five years. The exception to this statement is the median value of the CMAP-II surface for the right median nerve, which has not proved to be significantly different when comparing groups of patients with the metabolic syndrome and normal glucoregulation and groups of patients who had the metabolic syndrome and diabetes lasting for up to five years, although it was significantly leaning towards the neuropathic pattern when comparing groups of patients with the metabolic syndrome and normal glucoregulation and groups of respondents who had prediabetes as part of their metabolic syndrome. Since it is an independent sample, on the basis of that result conclusion can not be drawn in terms of nerve recovery after clinical manifestations of diabetes mellitus.

As for the value of sensory components of the electroneurographical parameters, they too were the highest in the group of patients with the metabolic syndrome and normal glucoregulation, and lower in the group of respondents who, as part of their metabolic syndrome had prediabetes; they were the lowest in the group of patients with the metabolic syndrome and diabetes lasting for up to five years.

Our research showed that the average value of all sensor parameters of electroneurographic analysis of median and ulnar nerves in the group of patients with the metabolic syndrome and normal glucoregulation were significantly higher when compared to the average value of the same parameter group of respondents who, as part of their metabolic syndrome, had diabetes lasting for of up to five years (p <0.05).

Thus, both hypothesis set at the beginning of the research proved to be exact (true).
The obtained results and conclusions necessitate the need for extension of the protocol for patients with this syndrome. The protocol would, among other things include the obligation of diagnosing changes in neurophysiological parameters in patients with the metabolic syndrome, regardless of the extent of glucoregulation. The aim of this diagnostic approach would be the early detection of metabolic syndrome repercussions on peripheral nerves, which would create the necessary conditions for timely and therapeutic treatment of the metabolic syndrome and its consequences to the peripheral nerves.

Early diagnosis and adequate therapeutic treatment of patients with metabolic syndrome results in preserving a high level of quality of life. This saves funds allocated for treatment and rehabilitation of patients who are primarily struggling with consequences that this syndrome carries.

It is important, but it is not sufficiently effective to conclude the state of neuropathy caused by the metabolic syndrome. Thus there is a possibility of multidisciplinary research in terms of the broad diagnostic approach and also in terms of therapeutic effect on the individual components of the syndrome. In addition to pharmacotherapy, rehabilitation and physical therapy is emerging as the main but not the only measure that can influence the prevention and recovery of patients from the consequence of the metabolic syndrome.

5 . Conclusions

1. In the group of 50 subjects with the metabolic syndrome and normal glucoregulation, there were two cases where the sensory response of the left median nerve could not be registered, and in three cases the sensory response could not be registered in the right median nerve suggesting that neuropathic changes were present in this group of respondents.

2. All sensory and almost all motor components of the ulnar and median nerves have been changed towards the neuropathic pattern in the group of patients with the metabolic syndrome and prediabetes, when compared with the group of subjects with metabolic syndrome and normal glucoregulation; the following values were significantly altered: the amplitude of SNAP to the left of the median nerve, the sensory conducting velocity and amplitude of SNAP for the left ulnar nerve, and conducting velocity in the right ulnar nerve. As for the motor components, those included the CMAP-I and CMAP-II areas for the right median nerve and the values of the terminal motor latency and conductive velocity for the left ulnar nerve, which leads to a conclusion of neuropatic changes being present, and more pronounced in this group of respondents.

3. In the group of 50 patients who as part of the metabolic syndrome had diabetes mellitus for up to five years the sensory response could not be registered in the left median nerve in four patients, and in the left ulnar nerve in two patients; in six patients it was not possible in the right median nerve and in one case in the right ulnar nerve, suggesting that neuropathic changes were more pronounced in this group of patients in comparison to the group of subjects with normal glucoregulation or prediabetes.

4. All sensory and almost all motor components of the ulnar and median nerves have been changed to neuropathic pattern in the group of patients with the metabolic syndrome with diabetes history of up to five years in comparison with the group of respondents who as part of their metabolic syndrome had prediabetes; there were significant changes in: the value of all sensory parameters for the left ulnar nerve and SNAP amplitude values for both median nerves and right ulnar nerve, and as for the motor components that is the case with the values of terminal latency of the right median nerve, the motor conductive velocity in the left ulnar nerve, as well as with the values of conductive velocity, CMAP-I, and CMAP-II areas of the right ulnar nerve.

5. All motor and sensory components in the right ulnar and median nerves have been changed to neuropathic pattern in the group of patients with the metabolic syndrome and diabetes of up to five years, when compared to the group of subjects with the metabolic syndrome and normal glucoregulation; there were significant changes in: the value of all sensory parameters both nerves, and as for the motor parameters that is the case with the values of the motor conductive velocity in both nerves, the implementation of both terminal motor latency values of both the median nerve and left ulnar, the values of CMAP-I area of the right median nerve and ulnar and CMAP-II area of the right ulnar.

6. Changes in electroneurographic parameters in the metabolic syndrome are more pronounced in the group of subjects with a greater imbalance in glucoregulation.

7. Sensory conductive velocity and SNAP amplitude are those sensory components that are more prone to changes in electroneurographical parameters in people with the metabolic syndrome; the most vulnerable nerve was shown to be the right median nerve.

8. The changes in the motor components of electroneurographical parameters in patients with the metabolic syndrome and greater imbalance in glucoregulation are more pronounced in the ulnar nerves.

6. Literature

Alberti KG, Zimmet P, Shaw J (2005) IDF Epidemiology Task Force Consensus Group. The metabolic syndrome a new worldwide definition. Lancet 366: 1059-62.

Alberti KGMM (2010) The Classification and diagnosis of diabetes. U: Holt RIG, Cockram CS, Flyvbjerg A, Goldstein BJ, urednici. Textbook of diabetes. 4. izd. Chichester: Wiley-Blackwell, 24-30.

Anonymous (1995) American Diabetes Association Consensus statement: standardized measures in diabetic neuropathy. Diabetes Care 18(Suppl 1):59-82.
Anonymous (1999) Definition, diagnosis and classification of diabetes mellitus and its complications. Part 1: diagnosis and classification of diabetes mellitus. Geneva: WHO Department of Noncommunicable Disease Surveillance.

Anonymous (2001) Executive Summary of The Third Report of the National Cholesterol Education Program (NCEP) Expert Panel on Detection, Evaluation and Treatment of High Blood Cholesterol in Adults (Adult Treatment Panel III). JAMA 285:2486-97.

Anonymous (2003) International Diabetes Federation. Diabetes Atlas 2000. Brussels; IDF.

Anonymous (2003) The Expert Committee on the Diagnosis and Classification of Diabetes mellitus. Report of the expert commitee on the diagnosis and classification of diabetes mellitus. Diabetes Care 26:5-20.

Anonymous (2004) American Diabetes Association. Diagnosis and classification of diabetes mellitus. Diabetes Care 27:5-10.

Anonymous (2005) Diagnosis and management of the metabolic syndrome: an American Heart Association/National Heart, Lung, and Blood Institute Scientific Statement. Circulation 112:2735-52.

Anonymous (2007) Ryden L, Standl E, Bartnik M, Van den Berghe G, Betteridge J, De Boer MJ, Cosentino F, Jönsson B, Laakso M, Malmberg K, Priori S, Östergren J, Toumilehto J, Trainsdottir I. Guidelines on Diabetes, Pre-Diabetes and Cardiovascular Diseases: Executuve Summary. The Task Force on Diabetes and Cardiovascular Diseases of The European Society of Cardiology (ESC) and The European Association for the Study of Diabetes (EASD). EUR HEART;28(1):88-136.

Arezzo JC (1999) New developments in diagnosis of diabetic neuropathy. Am J Med. 107(2B):9-16.

Arner P (1995) Differences in lipolysis between human subcutaneous and omental adipose tissues. Ann Med 27:435-8.

Assmann G, Guerra R, Fox G, et al. (2007) Harmonizing the definition of the metabolic syndrome: Comparison of the Criteria of the Adult Treatment Panel III and the International Diabetes Federation in United States American and European populations. American Journal of Cardiology 99:541-8.

Athyros VG, Ganotakis ES, Bathianaki M, et al. (2005) Awareness, treatment and control of the metabolic syndrome and its components: a multicentre Greek study. Hellenic J Cardiol 46:380-6.

Avogadro A, Crepaldi G, Enzi G, Tiengo A (1967) Associazione di iperlipidemia, diabete mellito e obesità di medio grado. Acta Diabetol Lat 4:572-590.

Azizi F, Salehi P, Etemadi A, Zahedi-ASL S (2003) Prevalence of metabolic syndrome in an urban population: Tehran Lipid and Glucose Study. Diabetes Res Clin Pract; 61:29-37.

Balkau B, Hu G, Qiao Q, Tuomilehto J, Borch-Johnsen K, Pyorala K (2004) Prediction of the risk of cardiovascular mortality using a score that includes glucose as a risk factor. The DECODE Study. Diabetologia 47(12):2118-2128.

Barada A, Reljanović M, Bilić R, Kovljanić J, Metelko Ž (2000) One year follow up in diabetic patients after surgical treatment of carpal tunnel syndrome. J Neurol 247(3):753.

Behse F, Buchtal F, Carlsen F (1977) Nerve biopsy and conduction studies in diabetic neuropathy. J Neurol Neurosurg Psychiatry 40:1072.

Bell CG, Walley AJ, Froguel P (2005) The genetics of human obesity. Nat Rev Genet 6:221-34.

Brown MJ, Martin JR, Asbury AK (1976) Painful diabetic neuropathy: a morphometric study. Arch Neurol 33:164-71.

Cheng D (2005) Prevalence, predisposition and prevention of type II diabetes. Nutr Metab (Lond) 2:29.

Clayden Jonathan, Nick Greeves, Stuart Warren, Peter Wothers (2001) Organic chemistry. Oxford, Oxfordshire: Oxford University Press. ISBN 0-19-850346-6.

Cummings DE, Schwartz MW (2003) Genetics and pathophysiology of human obesity. Annu Rev Med 54:453-71.

Dauble JR (1980) Nerve conduction studies. U: Arnihoff MJ, urednik. Electrodiagnosis in clinical neurology. New York: Churchill Livingstone, 229-264.

David L. Nelson, Michael M. Cox (2005) Principels of Biochemistry (4th ed.). New York: W. H. Freeman. ISBN 0-7167-4339-6.

Deen D (2004) Metabolic Syndrome: Time for Action. Am Fam Physician 69:2875-82.

DeFronzo RA, Tobin JD, Andres R (1979) Glucose clamp technique: a method for quantifying insulin secretion and resistance. Am J Physiol 237:E214-32

Donahue RP, Prineas RJ, Donahue RD, Zimmet P, Bean JA, De Courten M, et al. (1999) Is fasting leptin associated with insulin resistance among nondiabetic individuals? Diabetes Care 22:1092-6.

Dyck PJ, Davies JL, Litchy WJ, O'Brien PC (1997) Longitudinal assessment of diabetic polyneuropathy using a composite score in the Rochester Diabetic Neuropathy Study cohort. Neurology 49:229-239.

Dyck PJ, Karnes JL, Daube J, O' Brien P, Service FJ (1985) Clinical and neuropathological criteria for the diagnosis and staging of diabetic polyneuropathy. Brain 108:861-80.

Eckel RH, Grundy SM, Zimmet PZ (2005) The metabolic syndrome. Lancet 365:1415-28.

Fagan TC, Deedwania PC (1998) The cardiovascular dysmetabolic syndrome. Am J Med. 105(1):77-82.

Fazlović S (2006) Statistika-deskriptivna i inferencijalna analiza, Denfas, Tuzla, 27-31.

Ford ES, Giles WH, Dietz WH (2002) Prevalence of the metabolic syndrome among US adults: fi ndings from the third National Health and Nutrition Examination Survey. JAMA 287: 356-9.

Ford ES, Giles WH, Mokdad AH (2004) Increasing prevalance of the metabolic syndrome among U.S adults. Diabetes Care 27:2444-9.

Gorter PM, Olijhoek JK, van der Graaf Y, et al. (2004) Prevalence of the metabolic syndrome in patients with coronary heart disease, cerebrovascular disease, peripheral arterial disease or abdominal aortic aneurysm. Atherosclerosis 173:363-9.

Greene DA, Stevens MJ, Obrosova I, Feldman EL (1999) Glucose-induced oxidative stress and programmed cell death in diabetic neuropathy. Eur J Pharmacol 375:217-223.

Groop L, Orho-Melander M (2001) The dysmetabolic syndrome. J Int Med 250:105-20.

Grundy SM (2008) Metabolic syndrome pandemic. Arteriosclerosis Thrombosis and Vascular Biology 28:629-36.

Grundy SM, Brewer HB Jr, Cleeman JI, Smith SC Jr, Lenfant C; American Heart Association; National Heart, Lung, and Blood Institute (2004) Definition of metabolic syndrome: Report of the National Heart, Lung, and Blood Institute/American Heart Association Conference on Scientific Issues Related to Definition. Circulation 109:433-438.

Hanefeld M, Kohler C (2002) The metabolic syndrome and its epidemiologic dimensions in historical perspective. Z Artzl Fortbild Qualitatssich 96(3):183-8.

He Z, Rask-Madsen C, King GL (2004) Pathogenesis of diabetic microvascular complications. U: Defronzo RA, Ferannini E, Keen H, Zimmet P, (ed.) International Textbook of Diabetes Mellitus 3th ed., Chichester, Wiley, 1135-1159.
Hristova M, Aloe L (2006) Metabolic syndrome - neurotrophic hypothesis. Med Hypotheses 66(3):545-9.

Hu G, Qiao Q, Tuomilehto J, Balkau B, Borch-Johnsen K, Pyorala K (2004) Prevalence of the metabolic syndrome and its relation to all-cause and cardiovascular mortality in nondiabetic European men and women. Archives of Internal Medicine 164:1066-76.

Jarret RJ (1998) Is the metabolic syndrome a relevant entity. International Diabetes monitor 10(3):3-5.

Kanauchi M (2002) A new index of insulin sensitivity obtained from the oral glucose tolerance test applicable to advanced type 2 diabetes. Diabetes Care 25:1891-2.

Kershaw EE, Flier JS (2004) Adipose tissue as an endocrine organ. J Clin Endocrinol Metab 89:2548-56.

King PJ (2005) The hypothalamus and obesity. Curr Drug Targets 6:225-40.

Korner J, Leibel RL (2003) To eat or not to eat-how the gut talks to the brain. N Engl J Med 349:926-8.

Kostić V (2009) Neurologija za studente medicine. Beograd. Medicinski fakultet u Beogradu 2:353-72.

Kylin E (1923) Studien über das Hypertonie-Hyperglykämie-Hyperurikämie Syndrom. Zentalbl Inn Med 44:105-27.

Lee CM, Huxley RR, Woodward M, et al. (2008) Comparisons of Metabolic Syndrome Definitions in Four Populations of the Asia-Pacific Region. Metab Syndr Relat Disord 6:37-46.

Lee KS, Oh CS, Chung IH, Sunwoo IN (2005) An anatomic study of the Martin-Gruber anastomosis: electrodiagnostic implications. Department of Anatomy, Kwandong University College of Medicine, Gangneung, Korea 31(1):95-7.

Lorenzo C, Serrano-Rios M, Martinez-Larrad MT, et al. (2006) Geographic variations of the International Diabetes Federation and the National Cholesterol Education Program-Adult Treatment Panel III definitions of the metabolic syndrome in nondiabetic subjects. Diabetes Care 29:685-91.

Lupachyk S, Watcho P, Hasanova N, Julius U, Obrosova IG (2012) Triglyceride, nonesterified fatty acids, and prediabetic neuropathy: role for oxidative-nitrosative stress. Pennington Biomedical Research Center, Louisiana State University System, Baton Rouge, LA 70808, USA 52(8):1255-63.

Matsuda M, DeFronzo R (1999) Insulin sensitivity indices obtained from oral glucose tolerance testing: comparison with the euglycemic insulin clamp. Diabetes Care 22:1462-70.

Meier U, Gressner AM (2004) Endocrine regulation of energy metabolism: review of pathobiochemical and clinical aspects of leptin, ghrelin, adiponectin, and resistin. Clin Chem 50:1511-25.

Melton LJ, Dyck PJ (1999) Epidemiology. U: Dyck PJ, Thomas PK, ur. Diabetic Neuropathy. 2. izd. Philadelphia: WB Saunders, 239-55.

Miccoli R, Bianchi C, Odoguardi L, et al. (2005) Prevalence of the metabolic syndrome among Italian adults according to ATP III definition. Nutr Metab Cardiovasc Dis 15:250-4.

Moghtaderi A, Ghafarpoor M (2009) The dilemma of ulnar nerve entrapment at wrist in carpal tunnel syndrome. Clin Neurol Neurosurg 111:151-5.

Nogueiras R, Tschop M. Biomedicine (2005) Separation of conjoined hormones yields appetite rivals. Science 310(5750):985-6.

Onder B, Yalçın E, Selçuk B, Kurtaran A, Akyüz M (2012) Carpal tunnel syndrome and metabolic syndrome co-occurrence. Ankara Physical Medicine and Rehabilitation Training and Research Hospital of Ministry of Health, Türkocağı Sokak Sıhhiye, Ankara, Turkey.

Papanas N, Vinik AI, Ziegler D (2011) Neuropathy in prediabetes: does the clock start ticking early? Nat Rev Endocrinol 7(11):682-90.

Papanas N, Ziegler D (2012) Institute for Clinical Diabetology, German Diabetes Center at the Heinrich Heine University, Leibniz Center for Diabetes Research, Düsseldorf, Germany 12(4):376-8.

Perusse L, Rankinen T, Zuberi A, Chagnon YC, Weisnagel SJ, Argyropoulos G et al. (2005) The human obesity gene map: the 2004 update. Obes Res 13:381-490.

Peter HB, Wiliam CK (2006) Definition, diagnosis and classification of diabetes mellitus and glucosae homeostasis. In; Kahn CR, Weir GC, King GL, Moses AC, Jacobson AM. Joslin's Diabetes mellitus. 14th ed. Philadelphia: Lippincott; Williams&Wilkins, pp 105-115.

Petz B (1997) Osnovne statističke metode za nematematičare, Naklada Slap, Jastrebarsko, 327-328.

Pirart J (1978) Diabetes mellitus and its degenerative complications: a prospective study of 4,400 patients observed between 1947 and 1973. Diabetes Care 1:168-88.

Pop-Busui R, Sima A, Stevens M (2006) Diabetic neuropathy and oxidative stress. Diabetes Metab Res Rev 22(4):257-73.

Reaven GM (1988) Role of insulin resistance in human disease. Diabetes 37:1595-607.

Rodriguez-Niedenführ M, Vazquez T, Parkin I, Logan B, Sañudo JR (2002) Martin-Gruber anastomosis revisited. Unit of Anatomy and Embryology, School of Medicine, Autonomous University of Barcelona, Spain 15(2):129-34.

Said G, Slama G, Selva J (1983) Progressive centripetal degeneration of axons in small fibre diabetic polyneuropathy. Brain 106:791-807.

Santaguida PL, Pierrynowski M, Goldsmith C, Fernie G (2005) Comparison of cumulative low back loads of caregivers when transferring patients using overhead and floor mechanical lifting devices. Clin Biomech (Bristol, Avon) 20(9):906-16.

Shaw JE, Zimmet PZ, Gries FA, Ziegler D (2003) Epidemiology of diabetic neuropathy. U: Gries FA, Cameron NE, Low PhA, Ziegler D, urednici. Textbook of diabetic neuropathy. Stuttgart: Thieme, 64-79.

Smircic-Duvnjak L (2004) Patofiziologija metaboličkog sindroma. Medicus 13:151-61.

Smith AG, Singleton JR (2008) Impaired glucose tolerance and neuropathy. Neurologist 14(1):23-9.

Stumvoll M, Mitrakou A, Pimenta W, et al. (2000) Use of oral glucose tolerance test to assess insulin release and insulin sensitivity. Diabetes Care 23:295-301.

Tank J, Jordan J, Diedrich A, Schroeder C, Furlan R, Sharma AM, et al. (2003) Bound leptin and sympathetic outflow in nonobese men. J Clin Endocrinol Metab 88:4955-9.

Taylor BV, Dyck PJ (1999) Classification of the diabetic neuropathies. U: Dyck PJ, Thomas PK, urednici. Diabetic neuropathy. 2. izd. Philadelphia: W.B.Saunders, 407-414.

Thomas PK, Tomlinson DR (1993) Diabetic and hypoglycemic neuropathy. U: Dyck PJ, Thomas PK, Griffin JW et al, urednici. Peripheral neuropathy. Philadelphia: WB Saunders, 1219.

Vague J (1947) La diferenciacion sexuelle, facteur determinant des formes de l'obesite. Presse Med 30:339-40.

Valensi P, Atalli JR (1993) Cagant S and the French group for research and study of diabetic neuropathy. Reproducibility of parameters for assessment of diabetic neuropathy. Diabetic Med. 10:933-939.

Van den Hooven C, Ploemacher J, Godwin M (2006) Metabolic syndrome in a family practice population. Prevalence and clinical characteristics. Can Fam Physcn 52:983-88.

Vohl MC, Sladek R, Robitaille J, Gurd S, Marceau P, Richard D, et al. (2004) A survey of genes differentially expressed in subcutaneous and visceral adipose tissue in men. Obes Res 12:1217-22.

Vuletic S, Kern J, Ivankovic D, Polasek O, Brborovic O (2007) Metabolički sindrom u populaciji Hrvatske – kardiovaskularna multirizicnost. Acta Med Croatica, 239-43.
Witzke KA, Vinik AI (2005) Diabetic neuropathy in older adults. Rev Endocr Metab Disord 6:117-127.

Yang EJ, Chung HK, Kim WY, et al. (2002) Carbohydrate intake is associated with diet quality and risk factors for cardiovascular disease in US adults: NHANES III. J Am Coll Nutr 22:71-79.

Yasuda H, Terada M, Maeda K, Kogawa S, Sanada M, Haneda M, et al. (2003) Diabetic neuropathy and nerve regeneration. Prog Neurobiol 69:229-285.

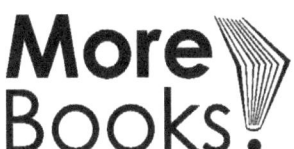
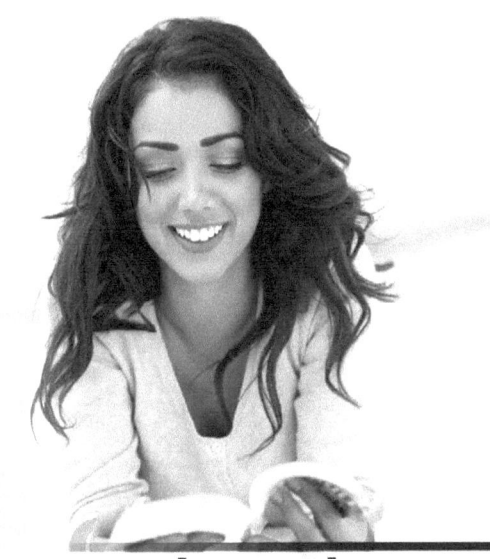
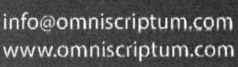
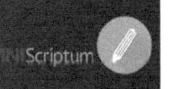

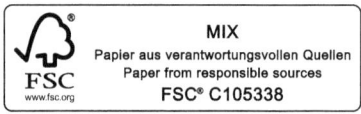

Printed by Books on Demand GmbH, Norderstedt / Germany